13 GREAT WAYS TO USE APPLE CIDER VINEGAR FOR YOUR HEALTH AND BEAUTY

...the essential handbook for Apple Cider Vinegar.

Alice Donald

COPYRIGHT

Contents

DEDICATION

This book is dedicated to God for the inspiration to write this life transforming book. I also specially dedicate this book to you. Yes, you for taking out time and the desire to change your health status and healthily as ever.

INTRODUCTION

The Apple Cider Vinegar has been known to be useful to man for many centuries. It is not just a recent drink that found its usefulness in recent times. It has been in existence for quite a number of years providing great uses and benefits to mankind. In this book, I have taken time to outline the great uses of the Apple Cider Vinegar to man.

Despite its recent surge in popularity, the extensive list of uses of the apple cider vinegar benefits has known well enough for quite an age. But only few persons are aware of its multifaceted uses. It has been known to be effective in keeping blood sugar level to the lowest minimum. Much more than this, the Apple Cider Vinegar has great uses in the health and beauty of individuals, most especially the female folk.

What the author has done in this book is to demystify the wonders of this commonly overlooked substance - the apple Cider Vinegar. In this book, you have a full exposure to the various uses of the Apple cider vinegar for the benefits of human beings in enhancing their health and beauty. This little book has so much value to offer the readers. You can't comprehend it all until you have a copy for yourself and loved ones. Inside it are great timely secrets to the potentials of the Apple Cider Vinegar. Do yourself good by clicking on the "Buy Now" to have a copy for yourself.

It is a complete compendium about the apple cider vinegar, hence making it the essential hand book for Apple Cider Vinegar as it contains all you need to know about it uses.

Wouldn't you rather get a copy and do yourself good?

With this book, you now have an edge in using an Apple Cider Vinegar. Get started right way by clicking the **"Buy"** button.

CHAPTER ONE

ALL ABOUT APPLE CIDER VINEGAR DRINK

Apple Cider Vinegar is also known as ACV. It is popularly referred to as cider vinegar. It is simply a type of vinegar drink that is purely made by the combination of apples with yeast. The yeast in the vinegar is to help in the conversion of the conversion of the sugars in the apples into alcohol when bacteria are added to the mixture. Apple Cider Vinegar contributes of 5%-6% of acetic acid.

As it is made from apples, it has some measures of water and minor amounts of other popular acids, vitamins and minerals.

General Health Benefits of Apple Cider Vinegar

The common health benefits of apple cider vinegar drink are found in the following:

1. For weight loss

2. Serves as food preservatives

3. For stabilizing and low blood sugar levels.

4. Healthy Cholesterol levels

How apple cider Vinegar is prepared

It is very easy to make Apple Cider Vinegar. It is not a herculean task. It is simply made by get apples crushed. When apples are crushed, then the liquid content is squeezed and served. To make the fermentation process easier and faster, bacteria and yeast are also involved by adding them to the liquid. Then the sugars are turned into the mixture.

Another phase of fermentation is also carried out, this being the second fermentation process. In this process, a conversion is done in which the alcohol is changed into vinegar some bacteria called the acetobacter. This Apple Cider Vinegar has a sour taste. This is contributed by the acetic and malic acid.

CHAPTER TWO:

THE USE OF APPLE CIDER VINEGAR IN BOOSTING GUT HEALTH

It is already established that the Apple Cider Vinegar contain some amount of bacteria. These bacteria are beneficial to human beings. They help in improving the state of your digestive system. In bringing about an improved gut health benefits to individuals, the apple cider vinegar makes the body to have an immunity system. Not only this, it also helps to give the body system an increased capacity to easily digest food nutrients.

CHAPTER THREE:

THE APPLE CIDER VINEGAR HELPS IN SOOTHING SUNBURNS

Do you spend much of your time under the sun? Does your work involving you actively doing tasks in sunny moments? You have no cause for alarm as the Apple Cider Vinegar is here for you to counter the effects sun burns will have on your body, most especially your skin. The Apple Cider Vinegar has been tested and proven right to be an effective substance in the soothing of sunburns. It is a great natural solution for the soothing of your dry skin. So, if you have skin has suffered from sunburns, all you need do is to combine a little quantity of apple cider vinegar drink with coconut oil, soak it and bathe with it. It is a perfect relief for your sun burnt skin.

CHAPTER FOUR:

THE USE OF APPLE CIDER VINEGAR IN REGULATING THE BLOOD SUGAR LEVEL

If you desire a good blood sugar level in your body system, you have come in contact with the right substance. The Apple Cider vinegar will satisfy your need in getting you a regularized blood sugar level. It does you great good by adding benefits to the level of your blood sugar. More so, it helps in increasing insulin level in the body system. To keep blood sugar levels stable, just take a diluted one or two tablespoons of the apple cider vinegar and drink before taking your meals on a daily basis.

CHAPTER FIVE

IT HELPS IN FIGHTING AGAINST FUNGUS

This is another great use of the Apple Cider Vinegar. If you want an effective way to fight against fungus in your body system, there is no other way to go than the way of using Apple Cider Vinegar. It is a proven and tested way to fight against fungus in the human body. You can easily treat all kinds of fungal infections such as toenail fungus, athlete's toes, yeast infections, and jock itch by the simple application of Apple Cider Vinegar. One of the most common and effective ways of using the apple cider vinegar is in the antifungal spray.

CHAPTER SIX

APPLE CIDER VINEGAR HELPS IN IMPROVING THE HEALTH STATUS OF YOUR SKIN

Apple Cider Vinegar is also found to be useful in the aspect of skin care. It has great applications by individuals aside their health. One of such great uses is in the improvement of the health status of your skin. If you want a natural way to improve the health status of your skin and keeps it ever glowing, the way to go is the way of Apple Cider Vinegar. It has great benefits to the skin ass it can help in the treatment of acne and to reduce scars. Apple Cider Vinegar is known to be effective with killing strands of acne causing bacteria. It is rich in its antibacterial content and healing characteristic, making it ideal to improve your skin.

CHAPTER SEVEN

IT IMPROVES CIRCULATION

Apple Cider Vinegar is also known to be useful in the improvement of circulation of blood. This also helps in alleviate symptoms of illness and diseases.

CHAPTER EIGHT

FOR TREATMENT OF WARTS

Are you tired of warts flocking all around your body? You want to deal with warts in a simple and most effective way? You've tried all you could and there seems not to be a solution in the nearest future. There is a solution for you with the Apple Cider Vinegar.

Here is what you will do: get a ball of cotton soaked in Apple Cider Vinegar. Apply it to the wart and cover with a bandage. Get this same process done repeatedly and you will see the wart falling off your body suddenly.

CHAPTER NINE

19

FOR HEALING OF POISON IVY

The Apple cider Vinegar is a natural reedy in dealing with poison ivy as it completely heals it. This, it does by helping in soothing the itchy poison ivy rash. This is made possible by the Apple Cider Vinegar as it contains potassium, which is very effective in reducing the swelling that is common with poison ivy.

CHAPTER TEN

FOR KILLING FLEAS AND BUGS

The Apple cider Vinegar is a natural remedy in dealing with common pests of dogs – fleas and bugs. If you have a dog that is constantly being infested with the presence of fleas and bugs, you can apply apple cider vinegar in dealing with these pests.

CHAPTER ELEVEN

REMEDY FOR SEASONAL ALLERGIES

Apple Cider Vinegar can also be used as a good remedy for seasonal allergies. Many people have found this Apple Cider Vinegar very useful in this regards as it has shown to work effectively in the lives of individuals. The bacteria in the apple cider vinegar are very healthy and beneficial. Hence, they have found a great use in the promoting of of immunity in the body against infections and diseases. They are also useful in supporting healthy drainages in dealing with seasonal allergies to a minimal level.

CHAPTER TWELVE

SERVES AS A GOOD DEODORANT

Have you ever sought for a substance that will serve as good deodorant for your body? Do you want a natural deodorant that works wonders? Then you have got the Apple Cider Vinegar at your disposal. The apple cider vinegar is a good and natural deodorant. When you have bad and foul smell as a result of the bacteria work under your armpits and other parts, the best and natural way to deal with such is to use Apple cider Vinegar. Since it possesses great antibacterial features, it serves as an ideal natural deodorant in excellently dealing with foul smells in your body. Just dip a tip of finger into an apple cider vinegar and apply it under your armpits in neutralizing bad odor and giving you fresh breath all day.

CHAPTER THIRTEEN

IT CAN BE USED TO MAKE YOUR HAIR SHINY

So there you have it! Do you desire to have a glowing and shiny hair? There is no better way to accomplishing this than using Apple cider Vinegar. Yes, Apple cider vinegar is useful in giving you a shiny hair. If you want a re-touch of your dry or full hair, the most effective way to do this is to apply Apple cider Vinegar on your hair. It helps in preventing dryness of hair thereby making your hair shine brighter, smell nicely and keeping it lustrous.

CHAPTER FOURTEEN
APPLE CIDER VINEGAR AIDS WEIGHT LOSS

If you are looking for an effective and speedy way to losing weight greatly, you can try out the Apple Cider vinegar. All you have to do is to prepare an Apple Cider Vinegar weight loss drink and see the wonders Apple Cider Vinegar does to your body in losing weight drastically. Adding it to your favorite green smoothie recipes will work better. You can try it out today and see the difference it does to your body.

CONCLUSION

So there you have it! Go out right away and start putting to test and practice all the information you have learnt in this guide about Apple Cider Vinegar.

Apple Cider Vinegar has great uses and at the same time have some positive effects on human beings. A great level of daily consumption of the Apple Cider vinegar has a great beneficial effect on individuals. Taking a controlled measure of the Apple cider vinegar will going a long way in propelling its positive effects on individuals. Strive to obtain and maintain the kind of healthy life you've always wished for yourself by taking Apple Cider vinegar.

Take a controlled quantity of the Apple Cider Vinegar and you will live a healthy live. I see you living well. You can check out my other books for your benefits. They will surely do you good.

Bye.

OTHER BOOKS BY THE AUTHOR

1. **DISCOVER THE SIMPLEST WAY TO MAKE APPLE CIDER VINEGAR TASTE BETTER**

2. **DISCOVER THE SIMPLEST WAY TO MAKE APPLE CIDER VINEGAR TASTE BETTER**